THE
ANSWER

THE
ANSWER

The book for anyone with ADD, ADHD, Anxiety, Depression, Insomnia, Autism, Bipolar Disorder, Epilepsy, PTSD, or Traumatic Brain Injury

DR. EDWARD CARLTON

Printed in the United States of America

Paperback ISBN: 978-1-947368-02-6
Ebook ISBN: 978-1-947368-03-3

LCN: 2017945211

Book Cover Design: ???
Interior Book Design: Ghislain Viau

To my wife, Paola. Her unfailing good humor,
and her willingness to see the good in everyone,
has made my life a better place to be.

Contents

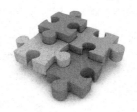

An Invitation to Discovery

Sometimes the answer to a problem is closer and simpler than you ever imagined.

Maybe you've tried to solve that problem with a string of conventional approaches, one after the next, that have left you disappointed.

But what if the opportunity to find a lasting solution exists just a *little off the beaten path?* Finding a better option may just be a matter of opening up to a new possibility—*an opportunity you haven't yet considered.*

That's what happened to me. I was a high-achieving health professional when, in mid-life, I was diagnosed with bipolar disorder, a brain-based condition that has caused great suffering for my family and me.

For years, I walked the orthodox medical path of trying to control my condition with medications. I took not just one drug, but many. Serious side effects meant more drugs, which frequently created more side effects. Some pills never worked; others stopped working over time, so my prescriptions were always changing. It felt like I spent half my life in line at the pharmacy. *And, despite all the meds, my condition did not go away.*

Then, by chance, I discovered neurofeedback training. Within a few months of my first session, my symptoms were almost 90 percent gone. *Even better, I was able to eliminate my medications!*

Neurofeedback training took my upside-down life and turned it right side up. My health, attitude, and the quality of my personal and professional life improved dramatically. Best of all, the training sessions involved no discomfort, no drugs, no invasive procedures, and little effort. As it turns out, with the right technology, it's pretty easy to retrain your brain.

Living a drug-free, symptom-free life has been a dream come true for me. I became a certified neurofeedback provider to help others find the same relief and reclaim their lives.

Research has found that neurofeedback training can benefit adults and children with a number of brain-based disorders, including attention problems like ADD and ADHD, depression, anxiety, autism, insomnia, bipolar disorder, seizures, traumatic brain injuries, and post-traumatic stress disorder (PTSD). Even if you don't have any of these conditions but are only looking to up your game, neurofeedback can help optimize your physical and mental performance.

This is my personal invitation to you to embark on the journey of exploration you'll find in this book. Learn how neurofeedback training works: effectively and permanently, with no pain, no invasive treatments, no drugs, and absolutely no side effects. See how these programs can be used to improve specific conditions or to optimize your personal performance.

Don't just take my word for it. Discover for yourself whether neurofeedback training is the right choice for you or a member of your family.

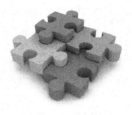

CHAPTER 1

When Medications and Therapy Just Don't Work as They Should

Modern medicine has brought tremendous improvements in our health, longevity, and quality of life. The development of antibiotics, for example, has allowed millions of people to survive what were once deadly bacterial infections. A child who breaks an arm on the playground can expect a full recovery, without any lasting disability. And today's screening and treatment methods have made some types of cancer completely curable.

But certain brain-based disorders represent an area where pharmaceutical-based medicine isn't as effective. Conditions such as ADD, ADHD, autism, depression, anxiety, insomnia, seizures, bipolar disorder, post-traumatic stress disorder

(PTSD) and traumatic brain injury seem to be much more prevalent these days, and they can be tough to resolve. The drugs used to treat them frequently carry side effects ranging from mild to severe—and from short-lived to permanent.

It's important to know that your doctor sincerely wants to reduce your suffering. The problem is that doctors typically follow established protocols, which means their "tool kits" of information for treating certain conditions may be limited. When you return to your doctor complaining that your medicine is causing constipation or dizziness, you're likely to walk out the door with an order for more medications to treat the side effects. These new medications might help temporarily, but they still don't address your true, underlying problem.

The Resistant Brain

The human brain is a natural wonder! It controls everything we do—awake or asleep, voluntary or involuntary—*and the vast majority of the time, it functions with remarkable efficacy.* A miracle of complexity, the brain is believed to contain about a hundred *billion* neurons (nerve cells) and a hundred *trillion* interconnections called synapses. Think of these synaptic connections as microscopic intersections. They are part of your own, personal, nerve-based transportation system for your thoughts, feelings, and action impulses.

These synapses are highly-sensitive junctions, allowing many things to happen. The pathways are both electrical and chemical in nature. When your heart beats or when you do almost anything else—scratch an itch, go for a run, fall in love, or study quantum mechanics—you are dependent on these synapses. *To think and function properly, the right messages need to be sent down the right roads to the right places.*

Given how hard it works to stay organized and the need for maximum efficiency, you can understand why the brain is a creature of habit. Let's say you've developed a routine of coming home from work each day, grabbing some snacks, and plopping down on the couch to watch TV or surf the Web. Every night, it's the same story. Once your butt hits the cushion, you're locked into the routine. It's like Bob Dylan sang: "You ain't a-goin' nowhere."

Maybe you know you need to lose the thirty pounds that are raising your blood pressure and causing you heartburn and back pain. Perhaps want to be more active. You might have begun berating yourself for seeming unable to get up and go.

But your brain resists, ingrained with that straight-to-the-couch drill. The more you repeat any habit, the more your brain reinforces the pattern, creating a "beaten path" using those well-worn synaptic roadways. Simply *telling yourself* you ought to get up and do something that will make you healthier doesn't inspire your brain to spend energy making changes. It's stuck in the slow lane.

7

So how do you break a habit? *You start by making a change in your routine. You do things differently.* Stop by the gym on your way home or go for a walk with a friend after work. Take up bowling or yoga. Sign up for a community college class. Whatever you choose, you avoid the couch and the TV remote at all costs.

Over time, shaking out of your routine teaches your brain to send its signals along *new* pathways. Eventually, you will have created some healthy, new mental habits and an improved routine.

The Problem with Mood-Altering Medications

Many brain-based disorders are resistant to treatment because of the same brain inertia that can keep you on the couch. For instance, doctors often prescribe anti-depressants known as SSRIs to treat depression. *These drugs don't change the kinds of obsessive, negative thoughts that can come with depression.* SSRIs artificially increase the blood's levels of serotonin, a brain chemical. This change causes the synapses to act differently, resulting in temporarily decreased feelings of depression—even though the underlying imbalanced brain patterns remain unchanged.

If the medication works, the patient feels less depressed and, hopefully, gets to enjoy an improved outlook. But this kind of treatment is somewhat like throwing a blanket over the brain to calm it down. The symptoms are subdued, but the depression hasn't actually gone away. *The brain continues to work in the same depressed groove, sending messages along the same synaptic avenues.*

Unfortunately, this is why changes in dosages and medications are so frequently required. The brain figures out a way to "throw off" the blanket, and the symptoms return. In the long term, the cycle will typically continue unless something is done to actually "change" the brain's routine.

When you take antibiotics for a bacterial respiratory infection, the medicine helps kill the germs that caused the infection, and you recover. The head congestion, sore throat, cough, and other symptoms that were making you feel rotten subside. In a sense, those symptoms were the by-products of the illness. The medicine targeted the *cause* of your illness, not its by-product symptoms. When you recover, you no longer need the medication.

With brain conditions, the only available medicines *target the symptoms*—not the source. There aren't any drugs that treat the functional causes of depression, ADHD, bipolar disorder, or other brain disorders. That's why we describe such conditions as being "resistant." Brain problems can't be eliminated like an infection, with a single course of antibiotics.

The drugs that treat brain conditions reduce the symptoms temporarily by altering the body chemistry, not by correcting how the brain works. *The worst part is that, if you don't take the medications indefinitely, the symptoms will return.* I was on medications more than twenty years for my bipolar disorder and was told I'd never be able to stop taking them if I wanted to control my symptoms.

A Better Approach

I found a better option that *changed my life*: neurofeedback training. Think of it as a fun, new "workout for the brain." This highly-specialized workout can teach your brain a new "M.O." and bring about lasting change naturally, without any of the problems you may encounter on the pharmaceutical road. It puts you back in the driver's seat, allowing you to take back control of your own future.

Consider my patient Susan. A college graduate and a successful businesswoman who worked outside the home, Susan was in her mid-thirties, married, with two children and a happy life. Or at least, she was happy until a few years ago, when she began suffering from an anxiety disorder.

Susan's anxiety worsened to the point that she could no longer drive, leaving her mostly house-bound. She stopped working and couldn't even shop for groceries or take proper care of her kids. She began taking anti-anxiety medications, but they didn't stop her condition from worsening. Her doctors kept switching her drugs and dosages, all to no avail. Susan developed insomnia, serious stomach problems, and other side effects. Then she had to start medicating the side effects as well.

Susan was miserable and at her wit's end by the time she found her way to me for neurofeedback training. Following an initial evaluation, I designed a protocol—her very own "brain workout routine"—to improve her brain function.

Just like going to the gym, changes in brain health take some time to work. After her first eight sessions, done twice weekly, *Susan drove herself to my office for the first time!* As she continued to improve, she worked with her physician to reduce and ultimately eliminate the drugs she had been taking for anxiety and insomnia. She cut the drugs for her gastrointestinal problems in half and, as of this writing, is in the process of eliminating those as well.

As you can imagine, Susan was thrilled that she could take care of her kids and live normally again. The neurofeedback training did this by helping her brain create new synaptic pathways to use, bypassing the old "anxiety roads."

Susan is finished with her sessions in our office. Since the training successfully created new pathways, unlike medications, there is no need for ongoing care. Her brain will continue to use these new pathways, further strengthening them in the future. *The result—no more anxiety issues!*

The Challenges of Talk Therapy

Mood disorders can originate in many ways. Physical trauma, such as a concussion from a car accident, can lead to anxiety and depression. The trauma of emotional or sexual abuse can create lasting changes in brain function that cause a person to constantly relive the abuse. Alcohol and drug usage can create short-term changes in how you think and feel, but they also can lead to long-term problems and a wide range of symptoms.

If you are seeking relief from these symptoms, counseling and psychotherapy can be an excellent choice. The goal of therapy is to create lasting change by helping you develop a new perspective on what happened in the past. In the hands of a skilled therapist or counselor, true healing can occur, restoring your control.

However, this approach can also be painful. It may require revisiting past traumas and talking through them in order to reduce their emotional significance. Depending on the severity and extent of the trauma, the process can take many months, sometimes years.

A Helping Hand

This is where neurofeedback training can help. Take the case of Michael, a thirteen-year-old adolescent who suffered sexual abuse between the ages of six and nine. He was receiving professional counseling, but the therapist was at an impasse.

When Michael was referred to my office, he was withdrawn, isolated, and struggling in school and at home. Despite the best efforts of his counselors, he was stuck. He hadn't shown meaningful progress in a number of months.

During his initial evaluation, his EEG (electroencephalogram) showed evidence of head trauma, which likely was experienced simultaneously with the sexual abuse. As a result of this damage, he was unable to respond properly in his therapy sessions. It was much like an athlete trying to play while injured: They may be able to get through the game, but they are unable to perform up to their potential because of the underlying injury.

Michael participated in neurofeedback training over a course of fifteen weeks while continuing with his regular counseling sessions. *I'm happy to say IT WORKED!* Not only did Michael experience a breakthrough, but when he left my office on his last visit, he was on his way to play baseball with his junior high team. *Confident and happy, he shook my hand and left with a smile.*

Neurofeedback Training: Change from the Inside Out

Neurofeedback training offers you an entirely different approach for eliminating many of the symptoms associated with brain-based disorders. It creates long-term changes in brain function using "operant conditioning." *This is a wholly*

13

natural process, with no side effects to worry about. If you've taught someone how to ride a bike, swim, or play a sport or a musical instrument, you've used operant conditioning.

Take riding a bike, for example. Your child climbs on the bike and you show them how to sit up on it without falling over, so they don't get hurt. Over time, they learn to balance, following your instructions and staying within the lines.

Sound familiar? Certainly it is! Neurofeedback training works much the same way to create long-term changes in the synaptic pathways we talked about earlier. These changes come from the inside and bring positive, permanent change, naturally.

Neurofeedback training is completely non-invasive; nothing is put inside the body and no dark memories need to be evoked. To the patient, neurofeedback training feels effortless. All they have to do is watch a video, and that's easy enough. As they watch, the brain is working and learning— using operant conditioning to improve its function.

With neurofeedback training, your brain learns to create alternative pathways for the chemical and electrical signals being directed by the neurons. The neurofeedback equipment measures brainwave output, using the results to create visual and auditory feedback for your brain to use in learning new pathways.

The feedback process prompts your brain to employ synapses differently. With no discomfort and no side effects, your brain learns and develops better, healthier neuronal pathways. These new pathways can create more balanced brain function, and—you guessed it—*the negative symptoms can vanish!*

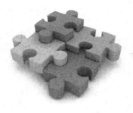

CHAPTER 2

What is Neurofeedback Training and How Can It Help Me?

Remember our example of learning to ride a bike? When you first started learning to ride, you probably had someone running next to you, holding on to keep you balanced. They probably said things like "don't lean too far left, or too far right, or you'll fall over."

The risks were there, because if you lost control, you crashed. But the rewards were also obvious. Once you learned how to balance, you were free to ride your bike by yourself!

A similar approach is used in learning just about anything—swimming, playing the flute, or even chess. This is known as operant conditioning, a learning system based on risks and rewards. The basic concept is that the outcome of your actions will either reinforce or discourage your actions; if you stay balanced, you get the reinforcement of a thrilling ride, but if you lean too far, you fall off the bike.

Operant conditioning is at the heart of how neurofeedback training works—except there's *no falling and no pain!* We use audio and visual signals to give your brain *subtle feedback* it can use in developing new neuronal pathways.

When you train your brain with neurofeedback, the brain learns new behavior. With time, the new behavior becomes permanent. This is exactly what happened once you learned to ride a bike. With practice, you grew more skilled at it. Once you've learned, the instructions became stored in your brain, and now they can be called up anytime they're needed. Unless you now have some physical limitations, you, as an adult, will be able to hop on a bike and pedal away—even if you have not ridden one for thirty years!

Remember that glorious feeling of successfully learning a new skill—like cruising on your bike without training wheels, or staying afloat and swimming across the pool? Suddenly, you just *got* it. You knew how to do it, in your body, down to your very cells. You no longer had to concentrate on the instructions. It became automatic—and it was fun!

With neurofeedback training, you can experience similar improvements in your life. Operant conditioning develops new neuronal pathways that tap into your brain's natural ability to learn new things, to organize information, and to operate better and more efficiently. Instead of bike-riding, neurofeedback can teach your brain new ways of operating and communicating to help eliminate insomnia, attention deficit disorder, depression, and the symptoms of many other brain-based disorders.

Your Brain is a Natural Learning Machine

Coaches in youth sports like to use the term "muscle memory." They teach players the skills they need to be successful, and then they have the kids drill and practice, over and over again. Some coaches even teach their players to spend time each day visualizing the process of smashing a line drive or scoring a soccer goal. The real or even imagined repetition of the proper techniques leads to athletic skills that appear almost automatic—as if the muscles *themselves* remembered what to do.

Well, it's not the muscles that remember—it's the brain. The brain controls the muscles and all body movements. When something is learned well, it's as if the brain wrote a playbook that it can draw on instantaneously and send out instructions, in a fraction of a second. An elite basketball player doesn't have to think about it as she jumps up, grabs the rebound, and tears down to the other end of the court, smoothly dribbling the ball in a fast break. That's because the brain has activated its miraculous natural abilities to learn, organize, store, and transfer data in the most efficient manner possible.

The brain has enormous capacity to store countless sets of instructions such as these—and then to communicate them instantly, as needed. You don't feel the neurons and synapses at work. You only feel the movements in your body that result from the brain's commands.

Certified providers use neurofeedback training in a safe and effective way that teaches your brain to galvanize its own natural learning resources, teaching it balance and helping it work more efficiently. Without putting anything into the body or making any changes to it from the outside, neurofeedback can—in many cases—*completely eliminate negative, brain-based symptoms.*

Although the brain's functions are highly complex, training your brain with neurofeedback is remarkably simple. As a doctor and former engineer, I could show you the math, physics, and feedback loops that are the "nuts and bolts" of neurofeedback. Maybe you'd find it a big yawn—or you might be awed by the intricacy and wonder of the human brain. But it's not necessary to understand *how* it works in order *to see it work for you.*

Despite the brain's complexity, with the technology we now have available, we can create a training protocol to improve your brain function using a qEEG (Brain Map). This protocol is a program to train your brain to do what comes naturally—creating and sending messages—but to do it more effectively.

When the brain works better, you feel better, because the brainwave imbalances that were causing the symptoms have been removed. The brain begins using different pathways that don't trigger negative symptoms. The problems that were caused by inefficient communications and imbalanced brainwaves have been retrained and fixed.

A Changed Life

The process can be quite effective. Take Marie, a professional woman in her thirties who had suffered for years from severe anxiety. She described feeling a grinding, ever-present anxiety that negatively affected every aspect of her daily life.

As a young woman, Marie experienced significant trauma. Unfortunately, despite drug therapy and counseling, she still mentally relived those horrible experiences every day, leading to continued mental distress. An intelligent woman, she had learned the coping skills necessary to live a productive life. However, happiness and peace eluded her.

Over the course of five months, Marie's neurofeedback training brought significant improvements. The repetitive thoughts stopped, allowing her to be calmer, happier, and better able to manage life's stresses and strains. Her relationships improved. Her coworkers complimented her on being better able to deal with difficulties. She became so much more effective at work that she received a promotion and a raise!

Marie was truly surprised at her brain's capacity to restore itself to a state of balance. Being a pragmatic person, she felt that the positive outcome of her neurofeedback training provided an excellent return on her investment. She compared it to the money she'd spent a decade earlier having LASIK laser surgery performed on her eyes. Her vision had been terrible, perhaps 20/200, and the surgery had corrected it to near-perfect, which made a huge difference in the quality of Marie's life. She'd had to pay out of pocket for the LASIK, she said, but she felt it was worth every penny.

After her neurofeedback training, she told me, "I want you to know something, Doc. The money I spent on the neurofeedback was an even better investment than the eye surgery. This has been life-changing for me."

The Story of Neurofeedback Training

Neurofeedback training has been in use for more than forty years, though its roots date back to the early twentieth century, with the first recording of an electroencephalogram done by Hans Berger in 1924. This discovery led to the ability to identify and classify brainwave types.

In the early 1970s, neurofeedback was first used to train the brain to better regulate brainwave patterns, reducing the symptoms of many brain-based disorders. One of the first therapeutic applications of neurofeedback was to treat epilepsy in 1972. Barry Sterman *eliminated* seizures in a twenty-three-year-old female epileptic, who then *came off medication and was able to get her driver's license!*

Over the past twenty years, rapid scientific development in the fields of computer science and neuroscience have brought important advances to the technology, knowledge base, and practices used to make today's neurofeedback training even more successful.

Measuring and Mapping the Brain

Before starting any neurofeedback training sessions, patients have what we call "brain mapping"—a measurement and assessment of the four types of brainwaves. The brain mapping process is as safe, painless, and free from side effects as the training sessions themselves. It's done using a qEEG, which stands for "quantitative electroencephalogram."

Today's equipment can measure every aspect of your brain's electrical output. Sensors placed on your head measure the brainwaves and send the information to a computer, where it is analyzed and compared to a large database of other brain maps. This analysis allows the provider to determine where your brain is going too fast or too slow and where any miscommunications are occurring.

The qEEG concept is quite similar to a fitness evaluation you might receive when you join a gym or hire a personal trainer. The trainer will run you through some basic physical tasks to determine which areas of your body are stronger or weaker than they should be, as compared to normal for people of your age, gender, and general health.

The fitness evaluation shows what areas you need to focus on in your exercise program. Maybe you need more aerobic time on the elliptical or in a spin class to build up your cardiovascular stamina. Possibly you're having back pain and need to strengthen your upper leg and abdominal muscles to take some of the load off your back. Or you might need a plan aimed at weight loss, to reduce your risk of disease and improve your overall health.

The fitness trainer performs the evaluation and develops what's called a "training protocol," a written document that has the details and timeline of a custom fitness plan designed to help you achieve your optimal physical condition.

The brain mapping that we do is very similar to a fitness evaluation. Because so many people have had EEGs, we have a very clear idea how the brainwaves should appear in the map of a healthy brain.

We compare your brain map to norms that are based on similar readouts from hundreds of thousands of people whose brains function more efficiently. These are standards derived from people who don't suffer from PTSD, anxiety, ADHD, autism, or other problems. Their brains operate within parameters that allow them to function without the kinds of symptoms that you want to eliminate.

During the analysis, we compare your results to these norms. Then we set a course of neurofeedback training to bring your brain into balance, to relieve your symptoms. Bottom line? *The brain map is essentially a detailed fitness evaluation of your brain.*

Pain-Free Improvement

Although there are many similarities between training your body and training your brain, there's one big difference. Let's say you're starting a new boot-camp-style exercise class, training for a marathon, or working out in the weight room with a personal trainer. You know you're going to expend a great deal of effort, and you'll probably experience some aches, soreness, and pain after the initial training sessions. You may hear the cliché: "No pain, no gain."

But neurofeedback training is safe, noninvasive—and best of all, painless. With neurofeedback, we can say, *"No pain, great gain!"*

Your Training Protocol

At the outset of a neurofeedback training program, I discuss the goals of training with the client. Using their history and the brain map results, we agree on the desired outcome of the training program. Similar to a workout plan, this program contains recommendations for the number of thirty-minute neurofeedback sessions, the overall span of time for the whole program, and the number of visits that will be needed per week. A training schedule will be created to reach the goal of helping your brain achieve an optimal level of performance.

The Training Sessions

Neurofeedback training can be done using several mediums. Some types of equipment use games; others use audio tones. The equipment I typically use features videos. The video itself is not the end point—it's a convenient medium that's used to focus your attention. You watch the video while the computer monitors your brainwaves.

When the brainwaves are out of balance, the audio and/or focus of the video are subtly altered to bring your brain back to focus. This happens hundreds of time a minute during a regular training session. It's not the video, but the continual refocusing of your brain's attention that teaches it to "stay balanced," much like riding a bike. By controlling the video and audio inputs according to the protocol, which was based on your brain map, we can correct your brainwave distribution over time. It works—just like a well-designed exercise program can make you physically fit!

Optimizing Your Performance

Do you have a high-stress job? Are you worried about keeping your job or finding a new one? Do you ever feel overwhelmed by the demands of your everyday life? Balancing the needs of your family and career is not only physically demanding, but also can lead to long-term brain fatigue.

Consider the story of Carolyn, a woman in her fifties who had worked in accounting for thirty years, even though she didn't have an accounting degree. Through no fault of hers, Carolyn's company was closing in a few months, and she was going to lose her job.

By the time Carolyn came in for neurofeedback training, the stress was getting to her. She was worried that her age and lack of formal education would keep her from landing a new job. She had substantial expenses, including a daughter who would soon be going off to college. She was so stressed and unsettled that she was presenting herself poorly and flubbing her job interviews. She was not performing well.

I incorporated what I learned from Carolyn's brain map to develop the basic protocol for her neurofeedback training sessions. She had an overloaded life and was stressed to near the breaking point. She was still working full time, conducting an extensive job search, raising a teenager, and constantly worrying about the future.

The patterns on Carolyn's brain map reflected what I'd call a kind of "wear-and-tear" on the brain. Regardless of the source of your problems, when you operate under high levels of stress for long periods of time, the brain can get tired. It begins to work less efficiently. This can negatively impact your mental state and reduce your performance in every area of life.

Carolyn's neurofeedback training protocol was crafted to bring her brain function back into a state of balance—and that's exactly what happened. Neurofeedback helped her improve her performance and ace her interviews. About ten weeks into her neurofeedback training, Carolyn showed up for a session, glowing. She'd landed a new job, and her new salary and benefits package was a 22 percent increase from her old job.

But that's not all. Carolyn was calmer, managing stress better and thriving in her new work environment. She was enjoying her job and getting along better with people. In short order, she was promoted. Now she has several people reporting to her, and is earning a six-figure salary. That's what I'd call optimizing performance!

If you'd like to dig even deeper into the literature on neurofeedback training, I invite you to visit the research page on the Carlton Neurofeedback Center website:

http://www.carltonneurofeedbackcenter.com/contents/research

You'll find links for specific conditions that respond well to neurofeedback training along with scientific articles, studies, and reports on the use of neurofeedback for each brain-based disorder.

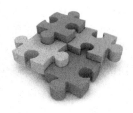

CHAPTER 3

I'm Not Just a Practitioner, I'm a Client—How Neurofeedback Training Transformed My Life

Even though it's painful to tell, I want to share my personal story with you. Why? Well, neurofeedback training gave me a new lease on life. The details of my journey clearly demonstrate that neurofeedback training can offer a dramatic turnaround for many brain-based disorders. *It worked for me, and it can work for you.*

Like many people, I've faced my share of difficulties. These include some major health challenges, starting as early as age five. Being a hard-working, outcome-oriented person, I haven't let my problems stand in the way of pursuing my dreams and achieving my goals. Today, I stay positive and

31

don't dwell on past troubles, except to apply any lessons to my present life.

After everything I've experienced, I know just how fortunate I am. I have two extraordinary young adult children and an incomparable, patient wife of more than twenty-six years, who is also my healthcare practice partner. My family stood by me with love and support during the past twenty years when life presented me with my biggest challenge yet: living with bipolar disorder.

To the outside observer, I appeared fine. I was working at my career, sustaining my marriage, and raising my children. In reality, my day-to-day life was sometimes very difficult. I was hurting inside, and my family was suffering, too.

I did what I needed to do—I took my medications, saw my doctors, and treated the side effects as they appeared. The conventional wisdom was that I'd have to get used to living that way, because I'd never get better. But I held onto hope and had faith that I'd find a better solution and resume a normal life. Ultimately, neurofeedback training proved to be that solution.

My Childhood ABCs:
Abuse, Bullying, and Concussions

I didn't have bipolar disorder as a child. It didn't show up until my thirties. As a child, I was hyperactive, the kind of kid who could never sit still for a minute. Looking back, it seems likely that I had ADHD. Attention disorders were known about in the 1950s and '60s, but they weren't addressed and treated as they are today.

I was born in West Virginia, where my family lived until my father's transfer when I was in my early teens. I suffered a couple of significant head injuries at a young age. Interestingly, those incidents were revealed on my qEEG brain map, decades later. The practitioner who analyzed my brain map recognized the signs of early trauma, even though I hadn't told him about my concussions.

The first head trauma took place when I was about five. My family was visiting a relative for a holiday celebration. One of my cousins brought the garage door down, and it hit my head and slammed me into the ground. I have no memory of the incident or anything that happened right after. My parents didn't take me to the hospital or a doctor. They put me in the car and we drove home, where I woke up the next day.

A year or two after that, I fell out of a tree while playing. Most of my memory for that day is also lost. Somehow, I made it back home. I recall my mother peering at me later that same evening and saying, "Oh, you're back." She then told me I'd fallen from a tree and hit my head, and that I'd been conscious, but in a daze for about seven hours.

I was just a little boy who didn't know anything about concussions. It was Sunday, which was the day we had pizza for dinner. All I cared about was whether we'd had the pizza yet!

We lived on a street where there were few boys close to my age. Those were the times before scheduled playdates and programmed activities—the days of unstructured free play, when kids would simply go outside and have fun. Sadly, for me, it wasn't always fun.

I was a small boy for my age, and the three neighborhood boys I played with were all older and bigger than me. Individually, they were okay. But when they got together as a group, they teased, taunted, and bullied me incessantly, both physically and emotionally.

Eventually, we moved away, leaving the bullies behind. The emotional scars remained. With the knowledge of brain functions that I've gained from being a neurofeedback practitioner, I can see that these incidents changed the way my brain worked.

Bipolar disorder has a strong genetic component, but there's more to it than genetics. What you inherit is a *tendency* to develop the disorder, not the condition itself. Real-world circumstances affect whether that tendency will turn into bipolar disorder, as mine did, many years later.

A Faulty Squat Rack and a New Direction

What happened to me was not unique, nor was the way I responded. I didn't ever want to be bullied again. As a young teen, living in a new state, I took up weight-lifting. And as another way of protecting myself, I developed an attitude.

As I grew bigger and much stronger, my anger kept me from getting along well with other kids in school, and I often got into fights. Nevertheless, I did well academically and graduated from high school a year early.

College was an easier time for me. I added power-lifting to my workout regimen, which gave me an outlet for my pent-up anger. Wanting to keep my temper in check, I also took a helpful class in meditation. I graduated with a degree in mechanical engineering and went to work in the oil fields of Texas, New Mexico, and Louisiana. I enjoyed my work greatly.

Things went well until an accident changed the course of my life.

I was power-lifting at a friend's house. One of our welder friends had made him a homemade squat rack—a metal stand that supports a barbell, allowing weight-lifters to perform squat lifts. My friend was much bigger than me, and we were working that day on our maximum lifts. My maximum was 500 pounds, and that's how much was on the bar that day. I wore a protective belt and used proper techniques to ensure safety. It was not sufficient.

The homemade squat rack broke, and then so did my back. The result was three ruptured disks and six fractures in my lower back. For the next four years, I lived with chronic pain, limping and using a cane. For pain control, I took Vicodin, which is a combination of acetaminophen and the opioid drug hydrocodone.

Although my job was physically demanding, I continued working. The intense pain, along with the long-term narcotic effects of the medication, led to another head injury. One day, as I was getting out of the car at the mall, I apparently passed out from the pain and suffered a concussion when my head hit the pavement. (I only know that because I woke up in the hospital later that day. A passerby had called 911.)

The turning point came about four years after my accident. I was in the hospital for two weeks of spinal traction, which wasn't helping. My pain was severe, I was heavily medicated, and on top of that, I'd caught pneumonia.

It was the eleventh day. I was lying there with the TV on when I thought, "I'm watching the Flintstones cartoon and feeling sad. How is this possible?" Something clicked in my head. I refused my next dose of tranquilizers and painkillers. Ignoring my doctor's protests, I checked out of the hospital and went home.

The next day, a friend suggested I see his chiropractor. I was miserable and desperate. "Yes, yes!" I shouted. "I'll go to Peru if that's what it takes to get better." A trip to South America proved unnecessary. Within about two years, chiropractic treatments had me up and walking, pain-free, and off medication.

During the recovery, I retooled my life in a direction I've never regretted for a moment. I enrolled in chiropractic school in Texas. My chiropractors had restored my health, and I wanted to make that kind of difference for others.

Bipolar Disorder Comes Online

So here I was, age twenty-nine, a student again—and loving it! I was president of my class all four years. I met the woman I would marry, and we made it official two months after we graduated together and received our Doctor of Chiropractic degrees. We moved to our current town of Manassas, Virginia and opened our chiropractic office as partners.

During my medical education, I'd begun to notice a few mood swings, but they were controllable. Mood swings are characteristic of bipolar disorder. But things were going well in my life and I was busy with my studies and my love life. My predominant feeling was one of thriving. In hindsight, I know the mood problems had been gradually increasing all along.

Untreated, bipolar disorder typically gets worse with time. Ironically, that's due to the same reason that neurofeedback training is effective. The brain uses neuronal pathways that lead to symptoms. As those brain functions become habituated, the patterns that cause the bipolar symptoms are reinforced and become automatic, like walking on a well-trodden path.

It's almost like the brain forgets there are other options, so it keeps doing the same thing over and over, blind to the trouble it's causing. Neurofeedback training uses that same process to reinforce healthier habits that are free from harmful symptoms.

Although my bipolar symptoms were getting worse, I thought I had them under control. But eventually, the time came when I knew I had to get treatment. I went to a psychiatrist, seeking help for depression. I still had not been diagnosed with bipolar disorder.

That doctor prescribed one of the standard types of antidepressants, known as SSRIs. I took them for about eighteen months and then quit. For a few more years, I remained untreated. It's extremely common for people with bipolar disorder to believe their condition is "under control."

It took family and friends to coax me out of denial with a dose of reality. Bipolar disorder used to be known as manic-depression. Its characteristic mood swings are described as "cycles." You cycle back and forth between the manic and depressive extremes. My cycles usually lasted about a week, but there were times when I'd cycle between moods multiple times in a single day. This can be exhausting and debilitating, not only to you, but to the people around you.

It wasn't until my mid-forties that I went for help again. This time, I had a diagnosis and medications that were appropriate, though not always effective. Over the years, I tried many different drugs, dosages, and combinations. The overall success of medication was "hit and miss." As the drug side effects and the complications of my bipolar disorder intensified, I needed more medications. I slept only about two hours a night. I had numerous physical ailments, including stomach problems. I even developed muscle spasms in my left hand as a result of one of the medications.

When I took the medications, I was calmer. The goal of this type of treatment is to take off the extreme edges—the manic highs and the extreme lows. With effort, I was able to work, help my patients, manage my businesses, and maintain my family responsibilities. Yet it felt like I was walking on eggshells. I had to cope with the mood-altering effects of the drugs, even when they were working, plus the side effects.

More than anything, I just wanted to be normal. The doctors said I would struggle with this unsatisfactory balancing act forever. But I never stopped looking for a better way.

Neurofeedback Training to the Rescue

The new era in my life began inconspicuously enough at a weekend professional conference. I saw a display with a six-foot-high sign promoting neurofeedback training and listing the conditions it could help. The minute I saw bipolar disorder on the list, I hustled over to learn more. They were offering a trial session. I knew I had to try it.

The trial was exactly like a regular neurofeedback training session, with one exception. They didn't do a brain map or design a custom training protocol. They used a particular protocol that helps calm brainwave imbalances in one area. Since it's not targeted to a person's specific disorder, the expected result is a general brightening of the mood and an increase in energy.

The demonstration was intended to give people a chance to see if they noticed feeling calmer and more balanced. I certainly did! I came out feeling alert and in a much more positive frame of mind.

It felt like the sun had broken through the storm clouds. I was still on my medication cocktail then, but I was eager to be free of my symptoms and side effects. I decided, soon after the conference, to visit the neurofeedback center that had offered the demonstration. I saw their setup and how they used neurofeedback training. I reviewed the reports summarizing their clients' results.

I made up my mind to purchase the equipment and start taking steps to learn the process. I decided to become a licensed, certified neurofeedback training provider.

I also began my personal sessions, with the goal of retraining my bipolar brain and reducing or eliminating my medications. Eager beaver that I was, I did my training in an intense manner—five sessions a week for eight weeks. After four weeks, or twenty sessions, I saw enough improvement that I felt I could start gradually weaning myself off my medications.

At the end of eight weeks, the difference was remarkable! I felt calmer and my levels of stress were much lower. I slept better. My mood was even and stable—gone was that "emotional roller coaster" I used to ride. I found myself able to respond thoughtfully to situations instead of reacting impulsively.

All the routine daily life activities that my bipolar disorder had made so hard were now easier. My subsequent brain measurements also reflected my subjective experience of the benefits of the neurofeedback training.

If my story sounds familiar to you, there's hope! It doesn't matter where the brain imbalances come from; neurofeedback training can work with the natural learning process in your brain to teach it new pathways. *The success I've experienced is not unique*; in fact, it's typical of the results people experience when they do the training.

Neurofeedback training was the answer I had been hoping for. *Now it can be the answer for you, too.*

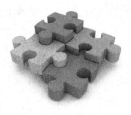

CHAPTER 4

What Actually Happens in Neurofeedback Training?

During their initial evaluation for neurofeedback training, people often share their concern that the process might change the patient. Naturally, a parent whose child has ADHD wants their child to have an easier time with learning, attention, and behavior. That's why they're sitting in my office.

But sometimes, there's a little hesitancy. "I love who my son is," a parent might say, "and I don't want him to be *different*. Will neurofeedback training change him?" This is a common question and, fortunately, one that's easily addressed.

The answer is a resounding "No!" When you develop a fitness plan and start a workout program at the gym, you may come home sweaty, but you're still the same person.

You may have more strength and stamina and better muscle tone. You might be able to run faster or carry your groceries more easily. You may lose weight and develop a rosier outlook. But you are still *you*—free to hold all your own individual values, beliefs, ideas, and emotions.

Actually, the disruptive symptoms of a brain disorder might be *masking* the real you. A student with ADHD may be unable to demonstrate their intelligence because of their inattention and hyperactivity. A person with anxiety may withdraw from social interactions and not reveal their friendly, interested nature.

Once neurofeedback trains your brain to operate more efficiently, you may find that your true personality— your intelligence, your ability to reason, your joy, your caring nature—can shine through in a way that previously wasn't possible.

Neurofeedback training naturally helps the brain find better, healthier ways to do its jobs. There isn't the slightest connection between you choosing to *train* your brain and what's called "brainwashing" or mind control. None! Whether in children or adults, the brain-based disorders we work with happen when the brain uses *suboptimal* methods to send information. Neurofeedback training helps the suboptimal become *optimal*, just the way strength training makes your muscles work better.

Think of an old, unmaintained road that's riddled with cracks and potholes. It's difficult or impossible to get where you want to go on that road, and you might damage your car in the process. Neurofeedback training is like a GPS that helps your brain figure out a well-paved, alternative route to get you to your destination, faster and more safely. But you are always the one driving the car.

The positive results of neurofeedback training come from inside you. They're not external. You can feel completely confident that your personality, identity, and all the elements that make up the essence of *you* will not be altered in any way.

The First Step: A Free Evaluation and Consultation

To give people a chance to explore neurofeedback training and discover whether it's right for them, I offer a free evaluation. (If you're reading this book and are too far away to visit my office, go to *www.bcia.org* to locate a certified practitioner in your area. The intake process will vary from one office to the next, but the basic steps will be fairly similar in most cases).

It's a straightforward process. When you come to my office, you'll fill out a form providing basic information for you or your child, telling us what your concerns are and how the condition affects you and your family. Parents or guardians fill out the form for younger children.

Next, we'll ask you to complete our online questionnaire. If you prefer, the questionnaire can be completed via our website in advance of your visit. I analyze those results before we sit down together. Then we go into my office for a private consultation that usually lasts twenty or thirty minutes. These can be one-on-one meetings, but people often bring their families with them. We welcome families at Carlton Neurofeedback Center.

Once we introduce ourselves, I'll invite you to ask any and all questions you have about neurofeedback training. Our goal is to ensure you have enough information to make an informed decision. People often ask questions like these:

- *What is neurofeedback training?* It's a technology that helps you retrain your brainwave distribution to reduce the symptoms associated with many brain-based disorders.

- *Can it help me?* That's what we'll determine in the evaluation. Neurofeedback training is highly effective for conditions that stem from inefficient brainwave distribution, but there are some circumstances where it is not the ticket. We'll talk candidly about whether neurofeedback might be right for you or your loved one.

- *Is it dangerous? Are there side effects?* I'm pleased to say that, in the forty plus years neurofeedback training has been in use, there has never been a reported case of side effects. That's because we're not putting anything in—we're just using the brain's natural processes to help it heal.

- *What's the time commitment?* Each neurofeedback session in our office takes thirty minutes itself, so we suggest you allow forty-five minutes per session. Patients normally come in twice a week, for a duration that varies with your schedule and condition. We're talking weeks or months, not longer.

- *Will I have to go off medicine before I start neurofeedback training?* No.

- *Will I be able to reduce or eliminate my medication?* That's very likely. We'll work closely with you and your physician to ensure a safe, appropriate process.

- *When will I see the effects?* Patients typically report that they start to see fruits of the training in six to eight sessions, which is usually about three to four weeks.

- *Will I need more sessions later on?* That's unlikely. The training uses neuroplasticity to create long-term changes in the neuronal pathways of the brain. Once established, your brain will keep using these new, more efficient pathways long after your last visit to our office. It's kind of like riding your bike; once you learned how, you just kept getting better the more you did it!

A Typical Visit

If you've reached the conclusion that neurofeedback training makes sense for you or your child, you then schedule an appointment for your brain map, or qEEG.

The brain map takes about thirty minutes. It employs a device that looks sort of like a shower cap, with tiny sensors that are the size of an eraser on a pencil. We place little dabs of a non-greasy conductive gel on the scalp first. There's no pain or discomfort. Typically, once the brain map or neurofeedback training session is underway, you won't feel the sensors and will probably forget you're wearing them.

When your brain map is done, we'll sit down in my office to review the findings. I'll show you where the brain map results correlate—match up—with the symptoms you're experiencing and the results of your questionnaire.

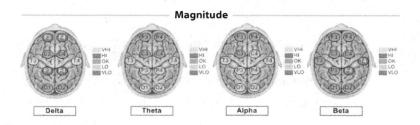

As this example shows, the graphical readout of the brain map makes it easy for you to see for yourself what's going on with your brain or your child's brain, and to understand how neurofeedback training can help fix the problem.

At that point, I'll explain my recommendations for your course of training—the training protocol. Your customized protocol will outline the advised number of sessions per week and the total course of training needed to optimally achieve your goal: to bring your brain into balance and eliminate your symptoms. You can then schedule your sessions in the way that best fits with your lifestyle and the goals of your brain fitness protocol.

The usual pattern is that your first visit is the free evaluation, the second visit is the brain map, and the third is your first training session.

What to Expect from your Neurofeedback Training Sessions

Most people find the thirty-minute training sessions to be relaxing and enjoyable. You wear the sensors so that we can measure your brain output in real time. Then you just sit down on a comfortable chair in a quiet room and watch a video. A parent may stay in the room during their child's session. We have a big selection of videos to choose from with DVDs, Netflix, and a full range of children's shows. In my office, I prefer to use positive types of videos instead of videos that include violence or negativity.

Your brain map has revealed the areas of your brain that function inefficiently, causing the troubling symptoms. As you watch the movie, the real-time measurements show when the brain is using those old pathways—like driving down that pothole-filled road. The mismatch causes the sound and picture in the video to grow dim. And here's where your brain's remarkable, natural learning ability comes in.

In order to keep watching the movie, the brain figures out it can exit the inefficient road and jump onto a new route—which it does! When the brain function switches to a better mode, the video quality is restored. This process is repeated over and over, which is why we call it a "workout" for your brain. It's not an instant fix, because it takes a little time for the brain to turn its new lessons into habits—much the way it takes repetition for your muscles to get toned and strong when you're working out with weights.

While many people don't notice significant changes until they've experienced at least six sessions, you may leave any individual session feeling pretty good. That's because you've just had a respite from the type of constant brain activity that can cause your unpleasant symptoms. Most adults and children find the training experience so enjoyable that they look forward to coming in.

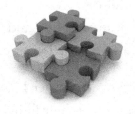

CHAPTER 5

"Look, Doc, Straight A's!" — What Can Neurofeedback Training Do for Your Child?

One of the toughest challenges parents encounter is watching their child struggle—day in, day out—with ADD (attention deficit disorder) or ADHD (attention deficit hyperactivity disorder). These disorders can cause problems for children in school, with their playmates, and in all their daily activities.

It's especially poignant when the child simply can't understand why the things that seem to come easily for other kids are so hard for them. They may have siblings who coast through their days, which makes it even tougher to for the child to cope with the reality of their own situation.

Among all the children I've seen in my practice, these two brain-based disorders—ADD and ADHD—combined, account for the largest proportion of patients.

Being both a doctor and a father, I hate to see the suffering this causes for children and their families. Providing neurofeedback training that improves the quality of kids' lives is one of the most gratifying parts of my practice. I get to watch the beaming faces of proud parents as their children tell me how their grades have gone up and how much happier they are. It's an endless source of joy for me. It doesn't get much better than that!

Consider the story of Maxi, a delightful nine-year-old who's been doing neurofeedback training for ADD. Maxi lives with her grandmother, who brought her to my office because she hoped to avoid putting the girl on medication.

Her school had recommended Maxi see a doctor for medication, since she had significant struggles at school, routinely bringing home Cs, Ds, and Fs. She had trouble focusing and concentrating. Although usually talkative, Maxi would clam up when it came to her grades. She felt defeated and embarrassed about her performance at school.

Neurofeedback training changed all that.

When Maxi was about seven weeks into her training, she came in one day for her scheduled appointment. She was smiling radiantly and waving something around with excitement. "Look, Doc! Straight As!" she exclaimed, showing me her latest report card. We were both thrilled—and so was her grandmother, who sat in the waiting room telling anyone who'd listen how well Maxi was doing in school. Well, grandmas have bragging rights, after all.

Children and Neurofeedback Training

The patient's experience of neurofeedback training is the same, whether they're a child, adolescent, or adult. The only difference is the videos they choose. We have a full range of kids' programming available, with cartoons being especially popular among youngsters. For small children, parents fill out the forms and questionnaires, but otherwise, the process is the same. We start with a preliminary evaluation where we answer questions and discuss how neurofeedback training can help with the child's specific challenges.

If they choose to move forward, we'll schedule a session for a qEEG (a brain map) and use the results to design the child's custom training protocol. We know some children are initially anxious about the brain map, and we reassure them that it won't hurt in the slightest. Their parents can be in the room with them. We are always careful to ensure that treatment is an easy and enjoyable experience for them.

Neurofeedback training can offer a welcome break in a child's challenging day. Most of our kids have disorders that

53

make school and activities stressful. A normal day for them means striving to meet adult expectations—sit still, be calm, pay attention, do the work, follow the rules, be nice to other kids. They feel like they're constantly being admonished.

We create a safe space for them, free of such burdens. They watch a cartoon and relax. They can't do it wrong and there's no way to fail. Can you imagine how refreshed you'd feel if you could take a half-hour break, smack in the middle of your chaotic workday? That's how kids often feel after their neurofeedback training sessions.

Neurofeedback Training for Attention Deficit Disorder (ADD)

Kids with ADD have a hard time maintaining focus, especially if their condition is moderate to severe. They have poor short-term memory. They lose and misplace things. They don't seem to listen when others speak to them, so oral instructions may seem to "go in one ear and out the other."

They have trouble organizing tasks. Figuring out the priorities and steps for the simplest projects can stymie them. Just cleaning up their room can be impossible. Understandably, they're reluctant to do things that require sustained mental effort, including schoolwork, sports, and group activities.

As it does with adults, neurofeedback training for children with ADD is designed to correct brainwave imbalances, prompting the brain to make new and better connections—pathways that better support sustained memory, focus, and concentration.

Nathan was a seventeen-year-old high school junior when he began neurofeedback training. He'd been on medication for ADD since age eight. Nathan tried neurofeedback training to improve his grades, which were in the below-average range, so he could get into college. He had always scored poorly in English.

After six weeks, Nathan's marks were already going up. When he showed his mother a B-plus grade on his English test, she thought it had been an open-book test. It hadn't. Nathan also experienced an unexpected benefit. He was an avid skateboarder, and he reported that increased concentration was helping him do better jumps, flips, slides, grinds, and other tricks.

Neurofeedback Training for Attention Deficit Hyperactivity Disorder (ADHD)

ADHD is another common condition I often see in children. As you can tell from its name, ADHD contains all aspects of ADD but with the added obstacle of hyperactivity. Kids with ADHD are always in motion—fidgeting, squirming, unable to hold still. They can be disruptive in class, where they have outbursts, interrupt, or get up and walk around the room. They don't always follow rules or respect boundaries. They lack impulse control and sometimes get into fights.

The medications for ADHD symptoms are mostly stimulants. These drugs help stimulate Beta brainwaves, creating better focus and concentration. However, that added focus frequently comes with a price: side effects that can include poor weight gain, disrupted sleep, and irritability.

Hyperactivity is a kind of self-stimulating behavior that arises from the brain's maladaptive effort to achieve proper balance. Stimulants quiet the symptoms, but they don't fix the underlying problems.

On the other hand, neurofeedback training addresses the *cause* of ADHD. The brain learns better ways to direct, integrate, and balance its functions. The processes that start all the trouble in ADHD are eliminated. And when they're gone, so are the symptoms of hyperactivity, inattention, impulsivity, lack of focus, and forgetfulness.

Teddy is a nine-year-old with ADHD. His mother brought him to my office after he was expelled from school because of his problems with impulse control and anger. He'd feel frustrated and afraid at school, and he often reacted to stress by hitting other students.

His mother saw a change beginning with Teddy's first visit, but the full neurofeedback training benefits weren't fully expressed for several more weeks. When Teddy finished his training, he hadn't had a single hitting incident in a month. Teddy was elated, as was his mom!

Autism and Other
Brain-Based Disorders

ADHD, ADD, and autism are the conditions I see most often among children in my practice. Now called "autism spectrum disorder" or ASD, autism has a wide range of expression. It includes a number of brain-based conditions, such as Asperger's Syndrome, which all fall under the ASD umbrella. The effects of ASD run from mild to severe. The condition can affect social skills, communication, speech, and other mental functions.

Neurofeedback training can be extremely beneficial for autistic kids, with positive responses on various scales that measure outcomes in kids with ASD. It's important to note, however, that the goals we set with autism are different than with other conditions. That's because the autistic brain never becomes un-autistic, so to speak. We therefore set realistic goals for measurable improvements in areas such as communications, behaviors, and helping kids to feel calmer and happier.

Neurofeedback training also can be effective for any of the disorders we've mentioned throughout the book such as depression, bipolar disorder, and PTSD. Those conditions are far less common in children than adults, but when they do occur, the child's brain often responds to the training as well as an adult's brain.

For example, my patient Allison had abruptly developed a serious case of insomnia. Allison should have been in ninth grade when I saw her, but she'd missed the whole first half of her school year because she wasn't able to sleep more than an hour at a time. She couldn't go to school, couldn't see her friends, and had to be home-schooled.

Doctors and specialists explored every possible cause of Allison's insomnia, but they were unable to identify its source. Her parents brought her to neurofeedback training as a last resort.

It's working! Allison's sleep is not yet perfect, but it's vastly improved. She was able to return to school even before her neurofeedback training was complete. Allison was tired of being cooped up at home for so long, and she was overjoyed to go back to school and resume the active life she used to have.

When Neurofeedback Training is Not the Right Choice

Most children do great with neurofeedback training—but there are some instances where it's not appropriate. For one thing, we don't see children younger than six years old. This is not because the training would hurt them or because they might not benefit from it. The main reason is brain development. Before age six, the brain doesn't have enough physiological maturity, meaning there isn't enough differentiation among the four types of brainwaves. That makes it hard to correctly interpret a brain map.

An easy way to understand this is to think about a baby. A five-month-old baby can barely roll over, but at a year, they're pulling up, cruising along while holding on, and maybe even walking on their own. At five months and a year, the brain's skills and maturity level are vastly different. By the same token, it takes until about age six for the brain to create the patterns that will show up clearly on a brain map to determine the best neurofeedback training protocols.

It happens only rarely, but sometimes kids older than six are not suitable candidates for neurofeedback training. The child may be so hyperactive that they literally cannot sit still long enough to have the sensors attached. The child might have a certain kind of sensory integration condition that means they cannot bear to have anything touch their heads, so we cannot apply the necessary sensors.

I always try to help the parents in these cases, and sometimes refer them to a doctor for appropriate treatment, including medications. In one recent case, the parents took the child to a psychiatrist for medications and returned to see me a few months later. Much calmer now, that child was able to begin neurofeedback training and has shown significant improvement in just two months!

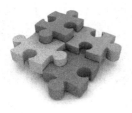

CHAPTER 6

Optimizing Performance with Neurofeedback Training

Most people familiar with neurofeedback training know it as a health modality that's used to fix specific, brain-based disorders and conditions. As awareness of this brain-fitness system grows, however, more and more people are learning that its uses and benefits extend beyond just correcting specific problems.

If your brain is functioning at normal or above-normal levels, neurofeedback training can enhance its operations, bringing improved performance in all areas of your life. Neurofeedback training can help you tune out the extraneous "noise" and calm the chatter in your head, allowing you better focus and enhanced performance at work, play, sports, and daily activities.

Increasing your brain's efficiency can help you improve *all* your skills, including driving, dancing, and even piano-playing! It also can help you learn more effective ways to manage the complex and stressful aspects of our modern world.

There's no difference between neurofeedback training for optimizing performance or for, say, eliminating depression. The goal in all cases is to teach the brain to work better. It's just the starting point that may differ.

For example, the brain of someone with chronic insomnia may be operating at only 40 percent efficiency when the patient comes to my office. Meanwhile, a person hoping to heighten athletic performance may already be at 85 percent efficiency when they walk through the door. Fortunately, neurofeedback training doesn't discriminate. Wherever you start out, it can help you achieve your goals.

And remember, they are *your* goals and *your* effort. It's easy to think of neurofeedback training as a passive activity, but just like with an exercise program, you're the one in control. Whether it's for correcting a disorder or optimizing performance, starting a course of neurofeedback training is another way to take care of yourself. You can use neurofeedback training as a tool to heal your brain and make it stronger.

Neurofeedback Training Puts Entrepreneur Back on Track

Jose's adult life is a classic story of a self-made man. By his mid-forties, Jose was CEO of a prosperous corporate-maintenance firm with hundreds of employees and offices in several states. Jose had a wife and young daughter, and he thrived in both his family life and his work. He was a dynamo who loved running his company, taking pride in his creative solutions and positive relationships with clients.

There's nothing unhealthy about hard work. To the contrary, if you like what you're doing, hard work can be a positive stress that enhances your well-being. But today, partially due to advances in computers and technology, many of us work grueling hours with little downtime from our work. We aren't able to renew and refresh ourselves in a lightning-paced business environment.

In Jose's case, the signs of work-induced brain fatigue were accumulating due to the overload. "Doc," he told me, "I've been doing this for twenty years, but now the success of my business is in trouble." His creativity was blocked. He couldn't find solutions any more. He was afraid to answer the phone. "I'm no longer comfortable dealing with clients, and that used to be my strongest suit."

The stress was bleeding over into his home life, he said. He was irritable and not sleeping well. "I feel frustrated and angry. I'm lashing out at my family, and I know it's not them—it's me. That's why I'm here."

Because Jose's "normal" level of function was very high, he was still able to run his business, even with reduced mental performance. But he wanted to optimize that performance and return to his previous level, when his work was fun and his home life was a pleasure.

Neurofeedback training was the answer for Jose. We worked out a training schedule to accommodate his travel needs. Instead of the typical, twice-weekly visits for a number of weeks, Jose came in five days a week for two weeks, with plans to complete the course when he had a travel break.

After those first ten sessions, Jose saw major improvements. When we talked, he was laughing merrily about the return of his creativity. "I came up with a great idea for one of my facilities," he said. "My idea made ten times the amount of money that I've paid you—and that's a great return on my investment! I'm answering the phone and talking to clients again. And when I come home from work at the end of the day, my wife is happy to see me."

How Neurofeedback Training Enhances Performance

When you consider the benefits of neurofeedback training, it's clear why this training can help optimize performance. Among the first changes people notice are improvements in focus, concentration, and the ability to sustain attention to launch and complete tasks. People tell us they have begun feeling more creative. They feel physically better, with less pain and fewer ailments. They sleep better. They're more refreshed and energetic during the day, which gives them a brighter attitude. Now that's a positive feedback loop!

Another useful, performance-enhancing benefit of neurofeedback training is improving both short-term and working memory. These types of memory are not the same. Short-term memory is information that's temporarily accessible to your brain for immediate use. Working memory is more like an operating system that makes it possible to retrieve and use information. When you improve both types of memory, you do everything more efficiently—from job responsibilities to homework to cleaning the bathroom.

Have you ever had a thought you couldn't get out of your mind? Perhaps you felt wronged by your employer or had an argument with a relative. Whatever the trigger, you might have had repetitive, uncontrollable thoughts about it, long after the stimulus stopped.

This obsessive or repetitive thinking is known in psychology as *perseveration*. The thought loops of perseveration are a major hindrance to optimal performance, because every time you focus on a task at hand, your mind drifts back to run that same old mental drill again.

Neurofeedback training can teach your brain to work smarter. It's like you hit the STOP button on the obsessive-thought tape player inside your head. The recurring thoughts stop happening, so you're free to direct full attention to the task in front of you.

Naturally, when your mental engine is firing on all cylinders—and pulling you forward instead of going in circles, remembering the past—you think more clearly and focus on the here and now. That's optimal performance.

Getting in the Zone

Runners and other athletes know the feeling of being "in the zone." When you're in that zone, your technique is excellent and your body and mind are harmoniously coordinated. You're certainly working hard as you log the miles or swim the laps, but it feels effortless and even pleasant. Your brain has learned the ideal pathways for the signals that orchestrate all the elements of the athletic activity. You may experience a "runner's high" when your brain releases hormones known as endorphins that create a sense of euphoria.

Elite athletes tend to get in the zone easily, because they have practiced and drilled to achieve high levels of strength, aerobic capacity, and technical skill. They've taught their minds to focus on their endeavor with pinpoint precision, tuning out any extraneous noise that might distract their attention. That's how a Major League baseball slugger, with a ball approaching at ninety-five miles an hour, can train his eyes to see it in slow motion, responding with a beautiful swing and scoring an RBI double—even in a tie game in the ninth inning of a playoff game, with fifty thousand fans on their feet and screaming!

Professional athletes often improve performance with neurofeedback training, and so can you. You don't even have to exercise regularly, though I encourage you to do so for your health's sake. If you want to improve athletic performance—whether it's for friendly weekend tennis games or competitive sports—there's no way around training, learning, and practicing. But by improving your ability to focus, neurofeedback training can help you train smarter and, ultimately, play better.

Stevie was a young teenager with anxiety and ADHD who came in for neurofeedback training. A multi-sport athlete, his passion was baseball. He dreamed of earning a scholarship to play ball in college.

After three weeks of neurofeedback training, Stevie's anxiety and ADHD began to improve—but what really excited him was how much better he became at sports. His mother said his coach was astounded at the difference in Stevie's performance.

Neurofeedback training had boosted his focus, concentration, and attention. The improvement to his athletic performance was one of the additional benefits.

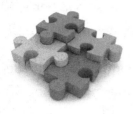

CHAPTER 7

How Neurofeedback Training Affects the Aging Process

If you're an adult of a certain age, you'll know this feeling. You're down in the garage, folding the laundry or vacuuming out your car. You go into the house, climb the stairs to the bedroom—and stop abruptly. Feeling frustrated and a little disoriented, you think, "I can't remember why I came up here ..."

You peer around the room, seeking something that will trigger the memory that has slipped to the back of your mind. Aggravated, you head back downstairs empty-handed, muttering to yourself, "I'm getting old."

Think how many times you've heard people meekly surrender to their deteriorating mental status. "It's just part of aging," they sigh. "It happens to everybody." But how does that explain people like actress Betty White, still memorizing lines in her mid-nineties for starring TV roles?

How do we account for John Goodenough, an engineering professor at my alma mater—the University of Texas at Austin—who at age fifty-seven invented the lithium ion battery? Now, at the ripe young age of ninety-four, he leads the team that developed the first all-solid-state battery cell, which promises huge advances in electric vehicles, mobile electronics, and energy-storage technology.

We see some people pushing a hundred leading dynamic lives, while others wind up institutionalized at eighty or earlier with dementia. If the destructive forces of aging were inevitable, surely they'd affect everyone more or less the same. Disease and genetic factors might account for some of the difference, but the discrepancies in the quality of life that different older people enjoy tell us that cognitive decay is not an inevitable consequence of aging.

Neurofeedback training offers the chance to correct or prevent the kinds of mental decline you thought you'd have to just grin and bear as you grew older. Please don't get me wrong—I'm not in any way suggesting that neurofeedback training is a "fountain of youth." We're all mortal and we're all vulnerable to inherited and environmental circumstances that can impact our lives. But just as appropriate physical exercise can improve your body at any age, neurofeedback training can improve your mental fitness at any age by increasing the functional efficiency of your brain.

The Good and the Bad
of an Aging Brain

The human brain is a sophisticated data storehouse. It remembers everything! The brain is immensely complex, but the ways in which aging affects brain functions are actually pretty easy to understand.

As we get older, our brains give us the capacity to expand our expertise and skills and to develop the wisdom we need to make reasoned decisions. Using the tools of emotional intelligence, we learn to stay calmer and more composed when dealing with stressful situations and difficult people. We even have the chance to become more compassionate, empathetic, patient, and loving.

At sixty, we may not have the strength and reflexes we had at twenty—but instead, we have a depth of wisdom and competencies that a twenty-year-old can't begin to imagine. These are the benefits of aging.

On the downside, getting older makes us creatures of habit. There are compelling evolutionary reasons why the brain likes habitual behaviors. Early humans who learned a new technique were far better off if they could remember and teach it, rather than having to figure out a strategy all over again each time they took up the task.

The problem is that a brain accustomed to routine has less flexibility—less *neuroplasticity*. That quality, as we have mentioned, is the brain's ability to form *new* neural connections. We need neuroplasticity to heal from injury, respond to new situations, or develop healthier mental habits. In terms of daily life activities, having less neuroplasticity means you are more likely to do the same things over and over—even when you'd be better served by responding differently, using other neuronal pathways.

They say you "can't teach an old dog new tricks." In reality, you *can* teach the human brain new tricks, as we see in my office every day—with neurofeedback training.

When your brain reacts habitually, it's sending signals along those well-worn neuronal pathways. Habitual thinking can be helpful at times. For instance, let's say you've become so expert at knitting that your fingers work the needles and yarn automatically, allowing you to knit without thinking while you're riding the bus to work. "Autopilot thinking" can be great for a craft like knitting, but it also creates expectations based on what has happened before—not what is happening now. Autopilot can become an obstacle when you're thrust into a brand-new situation.

A few years ago, a photo of a striped dress went viral all over the Internet. Due to odd lighting and variations in individual color perception, some people saw the dress as white and gold, while to others it looked blue and black. People engaged in heated arguments and scientific debate on the issues.

But "The Dress" issue also pointed out something important about brain flexibility. People who *first* saw the dress as white and gold found it difficult or impossible to see it as blue and black. Like a library book shelved with Dewey Decimal System codes, your brain tagged that memory as a white and gold dress and shelved it in what it thought was the right place. The next time you saw the photo, even with different lighting, your brain recognized it and pulled up the stored memory.

Stored perceptions are efficient for dealing with the myriad routine tasks we do each day. As we advance in years, our "library" of perceptions grows, giving us instant access to an enormous knowledge base. Again, that's the upside of how aging affects the brain. The drawback is that you're always getting a book that you've already read, making it harder to learn new things.

Neurofeedback training helps you find the right balance, ensuring that your brain doesn't persistently use old pathways when they do you more harm than good.

Neurofeedback Training Makes Your Brain More Flexible

You don't have to accept mental decline as a normal part of aging. Memory lapses and other signs of cognitive decline can be improved with neurofeedback training. But it's important to remember that brain health doesn't happen in a vacuum.

Neurofeedback training is a brain fitness program. To sustain its benefits, you need to take proper care of your whole self. That means getting relevant medical care for any conditions such as diabetes, heart disease, high blood pressure, substance abuse, or obesity. And it also means making good lifestyle choices including exercising, eating well, and getting enough sleep.

A nice bonus of doing neurofeedback training for aging-brain issues is that it can simultaneously help you make those lifestyle changes you've been struggling with for so long. Neurofeedback training *can* teach that "old dog" some new tricks, restoring more balanced brainwave patterns and training the brain to use better and more efficient neural connections. This can help you bypass the old pathways that were causing your worrisome symptoms and keeping you locked in bad habits.

Remember, neurofeedback training can't turn back the biological clock, especially if you already have a number of disease processes at work. Rather, neurofeedback training shows the brain how to function more efficiently within the parameters of your present physical and mental status. Because the brain has vast resources, even as it ages, the outcomes I've seen in using it for aging issues have been excellent.

Joanne is one of my patients who enjoyed great results. She had a relatively healthy life when her daughter brought her in to see me. At age ninety-four, Joanne lived alone, doing her own shopping, cooking, and daily activities. She came in for neurofeedback training because cognitive decline was threatening her independence.

Joanne had noticed that she was starting to have trouble remembering words and expressing herself. She sometimes forgot people's names and faces. She'd head out somewhere, forget where she was going, and then grow confused and disoriented.

Joanne noticed significant improvement after her first twenty neurofeedback sessions and was extremely pleased by the time she completed her course of training. She'd been fearful about winding up in a nursing home, but now felt much more comfortable in her independent life. Joanne could express herself again, using the words she needed. She remembered people's names and faces, as well as her connections to them. She could go to the market, complete her shopping, and return home without any confusion or forgetfulness.

Getting Out in Front of the Problem

Most people know by now that, if they hope to prevent heart disease, stroke, and other diseases associated with aging, they need to develop healthy habits. They need to watch their diets, quit smoking, and reduce their stress—as well as participating in regular exercise. This is particularly true if the disease runs in their family. Obviously, it's better to try to reduce your risk *before* a heart attack rather than trying to heal *after* you've had one.

The same concept applies to neurofeedback training. It's best to get the brain functioning in an optimal and balanced way to slow down the impact of aging before negative changes start to occur.

People interested in keeping their brain in shape to prevent cognitive decline typically come in for neurofeedback training when they're in their fifties. Training protocols can be designed to use neurofeedback in a preventive way. For example, someone who's fifty might come in for twenty sessions over ten weeks, and then come back ten years later for another round. This kind of training regimen can help maintain brain efficiency over a long period.

I also have patients who complete a round of training and then come back for occasional "tune-up" sessions, at intervals ranging from once a month to once every three months. The tune-up approach is helpful because, as they say, *life happens*. You might get your brain in shape with a course of neurofeedback training, and then life pitches a curve ball—a death in the family, divorce, job loss, money problems. Life has no shortage of stressors.

In the same way you have your car serviced to keep it running optimally, you can tune up your brain with a maintenance schedule of neurofeedback training that helps keep *it* running optimally—even amid life's changing circumstances.

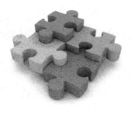

CHAPTER 8

If Neurofeedback Training Is so Great, Why Haven't I Heard of It
(and Why Won't My Insurance Cover It)?

Now that you've learned how effectively neurofeedback training works for many common brain-based disorders, you may be wondering about a few things. Why isn't neurofeedback training a frontline offering for conditions such as ADHD, depression, and PTSD? How come you haven't heard of it before? And why isn't it covered by your health insurance?

The answers are uncomplicated, though they deal with a complex system. They involve the way health care in our country is developed, paid for, and provided to patients.

Before we explore the subject, let's acknowledge what an excellent overall health care system we have in our country today. Over the past hundred years, huge strides in medicine and technology have brought major improvements in health and longevity.

I don't wish to disparage the care, medicines, devices, and procedures that have done so much to increase our quality of life. Personally, I have reason to appreciate our health system. If I had broken my back a couple of centuries earlier, the odds are I'd never have walked again—and that's assuming I survived the accident at all.

Resistance to Change

As to why modern medicine hasn't yet embraced neurofeedback training, consider what you learned in the chapter about flexibility and the aging brain. In growing older, you gain wisdom, maturity, and experience. You learn good ways of relating to people and solving problems. As your brain is learning these things, it repeats the same processes over and over, becoming more inflexible and close-minded. Aging becomes a process of contrasts, pitting positives against negatives. You grow older and wiser, but you also probably become more set in your ways and resistant to change.

Our medical system actually faces a similar dilemma. Over time, the system's knowledge and expertise has multiplied many times over, expanding its capacity to help people live healthier, longer lives. Yet those very successes reinforce the processes that led to the achievements. And, as Shakespeare wrote, "there's the rub." In a way, you could say that as the medical system improves with age, it's also growing more resistant to change.

Take physicians as an example. They receive superb training—up to thirteen years of top-notch medical education. They work intensely to gain the tools and expertise of sound medical practice in order to best serve their patients. By the time they begin practicing, doctors are experts, having amassed a wealth of medical knowledge. Clearly, that's one of the great advantages of a stable, established system. We get the best-educated doctors using the best tools in the best medical facilities.

Some innovation is built into the medical-education system, so that new drugs, devices, and procedures are constantly being developed and introduced. But innovation only emerges from *inside* the system, within the existing medical purview. Physicians use the available tools in the way they were taught to use them, and medical schools continue to train their students this way. Hospitals, nursing homes, and other allied medical institutions also function inside the bounds of accepted medical conventions.

This closed loop has many benefits, but embracing outside-the-box thinking is not usually one of them. Medical professionals often view anything that arises outside the loop with skepticism.

Although neurofeedback training has been proven to be safe and effective, it's not taught in medical schools. Pharmaceutical companies pour millions of dollars into research, development, and advertising of new drugs because successful medications offer a huge return on investment for those corporations.

By comparison, neurofeedback studies are smaller in scale, even though there has been extensive, quality research validating its benefits. The network of local neurofeedback providers is small in scale and doesn't have the kind of resources that medical companies can spend on massive advertising and physician-education campaigns.

Returning to the question: Why have you not heard about neurofeedback training until now? The bottom line is, most doctors are uneducated about it. That's not because they don't want to help you in the best way possible. It's because neurofeedback training was not part of their *allopathic* medical training.

By definition, *allopathic medicine* means using external agents, such as medications and surgery, to help the body heal. Neurofeedback training, which teaches the brain to heal itself, represents a more holistic approach. As such, neurofeedback is "outside the box"—and not yet on the radar of most allopathic doctors.

But that's starting to change, thanks to the many positive reports from satisfied neurofeedback training clients. In my practice, the number of referrals from physicians, psychiatrists, and therapists continues to increase as word gets out.

A psychiatrist recently sent a nine-year-old to my office. The child was on two medications and the parents were hoping to find drug-free alternatives. The doctor felt comfortable with the referral because he happened to have another patient who'd improved greatly after coming to me for neurofeedback training. This kind of referral shows the positive reinforcement of patients getting positive results.

Health Insurance and Neurofeedback Training

Referrals will continue to grow as the good news gets around about the safety and many benefits of neurofeedback training. What's unlikely to change in the foreseeable future is insurance coverage. There are essentially no insurance plans that will cover neurofeedback training. The economic structure of the health insurance industry generally results in restrictive policies that prioritize short-term savings over health benefits.

For example, if you were overweight and had high cholesterol and a family history of heart disease, you might go on cholesterol-reducing medications, or you might decide to join a gym to try to reduce your risk level.

The proven beneficial effects of weight loss and exercise in reducing cardiovascular disease risk are well-established in the medical literature. Yet cholesterol medications are covered by insurance while gym membership is not. Once you have a heart attack, insurance will pay for one-on-one physical therapy and the lifetime of medications you may require—but insurance is not structured to help you prevent that heart attack.

Insurance is a business of odds-making and actuarial tables. On a large scale, the insurance industry's coverage decisions may be helpful in providing the most basic coverage to a large number of people. That's primarily a good thing, since most of us don't have deep enough pockets to pay the exorbitant costs of routine care, much less the cost of other common medical events such as childbirth, surgery, or cancer treatment.

But we're not all peas in a pod. Health consumers must be well-informed in order to make the choices that best serve their family's unique health needs. Often, their choices to improve long-range health will not be covered by their insurance, even if they have a good policy.

Neurofeedback and Financing

After suffering for decades with bipolar disorder and dealing with multiple medications and their side effects, I found neurofeedback training. As you now know, this turned my life around completely. The relief it brought me from debilitating symptoms and side effects motivated me to become a provider, so that I could help others make their lives better, too.

My office accepts a wide range of payments and provides financing for those who need it. I don't wish to turn away anyone who might benefit from neurofeedback training, because I don't want to deny them the vast improvements in their quality of life.

In addition to direct payments, my office accepts HSAs (Health Savings Accounts), MSAs (Medical Savings Accounts), and FSAs (Flexible Spending Arrangements). We also accept the CareCredit healthcare credit card. If none of these is available to you, my office offers zero-rate financing and a payment plan. We want to help you feel better and we'll work with you to find a way to make it happen!

Neurofeedback practitioners in your area may offer similar, affordable options. If you are looking for neurofeedback training in other parts of the country, visit www.bcia.org to locate certified neurofeedback practitioners closer to home.

The financial realities of health care and insurance make it important for you to seek out providers who offer low-cost financing and a variety of payment options. Discussing financial issues openly and up front will ease any concerns and get you on your way to a healthier brain with neurofeedback training.

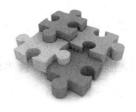

CHAPTER 9

Should You Try Neurofeedback Training?

This in-depth exploration of neurofeedback training was written to provide you with the tools you need to make a well-informed decision about whether to pursue training for yourself or a family member. You've learned how neurofeedback training works, how it retrains the brain to correct brainwave imbalances, and how it can help relieve the troublesome symptoms of brain-based disorders. And you've read many stories of people—including me—who have found relief from their suffering with neurofeedback.

Now that you have a fuller understanding of this powerful brain-fitness system, let's take a closer look at the steps needed to get started in my office. Knowing exactly what to expect can help you determine the answer to the question, "Should I try neurofeedback training?"

I've broken out the steps to paint a clear picture, but it's actually a pretty swift process.

Step One: Making the First Appointment

One thing you won't learn from a book is whether neurofeedback training is a good match for the unique needs and circumstances of your own personal situation. To find out, contact the Carlton Neurofeedback Center and schedule a free initial evaluation. Whether you call by phone or connect with us online, we'll get you rolling to schedule a convenient appointment time.

For those who don't live near my office in northern Virginia, I encourage you to find a certified neurofeedback training provider closer to home. You can visit the Website www.bcia.org and click on the "Find a Practitioner" tab. Then follow the steps to locate a neurofeedback practitioner in your area. Look for the letters BCN, which tells you the provider is professionally certified in neurofeedback training.

Step Two: Completing the Questionnaire

When you contact my office, we'll gather some basic information that will allow us to create a login that you can use to complete an online questionnaire. That's usually done in advance of the initial evaluation appointment. But if you prefer, you can arrange to do it in our office, even on the same day as your evaluation. It takes about twenty minutes. Parents fill out the questionnaires for younger children.

The questionnaire comes in three parts and covers many physical and mental symptoms that you or your child may have experienced, as well as the problem for which you're seeking help. Before we sit down together, I will analyze the questionnaire data. The resulting profile provides an initial assessment of brainwave distribution patterns that will later be correlated with the actual brain map.

Step Three: The Initial Evaluation

I offer a free initial evaluation in my office. It can be a one-on-one meeting or you can bring family members. If the neurofeedback training is for a child, they should attend. This is our chance to review the questionnaire findings and for you to ask me any and all questions you may have. The evaluations typically last twenty or thirty minutes, but I am happy to take longer in order to address all your concerns.

By the end of the initial evaluation, you'll have a much better sense of whether neurofeedback training might be an appropriate and helpful choice for you. Most clients then proceed to the next step and schedule an appointment for their brain map. A few prefer to go home and give it more thought before deciding to start. Either approach is fine with us!

Step Four: The Brain Map

The brain mapping itself takes half an hour. As noted earlier, it's an easy and pleasant process. Afterwards, I'll sit down with you again, this time to discuss the findings and my recommendations for a training protocol—your personalized brain-fitness program. Whether the neurofeedback is for you or for a child, we'll talk about goals for the training, finances, and timing of the sessions. This is another decision point in the process. If you're comfortable, you choose to go forward with the training sessions, so you can start thinking and feeling better!

Step Five: Gentlemen and Ladies— Start Your Trainings

This is the best part. You or your child get a respite from work or school to come in for an enjoyable half hour spent training, while watching a video. Since most patients start seeing some improvements within just a few sessions, the trainings become something they anticipate with pleasure.

We can work with you on a training schedule that fits the demands of your busy life. If you're a college student home on a break, we can accelerate the schedule. Going on a business trip? We'll resume the sessions when you return.

Neurofeedback Training: It's Your Call

When you come to our office for an evaluation, we will answer all your questions about your specific situation in order to assist with your decision process. But we will never pressure you. We respect your conclusions and want you to be comfortable with the process.

Neurofeedback training is not a one-size-fits-all proposition. Everyone is different. Your brain, symptoms, and training protocol—as well as your goals and desires with regard to the training—are yours alone. It has to be a good fit for *you*.

What happens if you reach your goals ahead of schedule? I will be evaluating your progress in an active way in every session. If you attain your goals before the protocol is complete, I'll happily suggest you wrap up early. You only pay for the services you receive. That hasn't happened with any of my clients, however. They're generally so thrilled with their progress that they continue working toward optimizing their full potential!

Pathway to a Better Life

As a provider, it's been a joy and a privilege to use this technology to help people overcome brain-based disorders. I've seen many patients enhance their performance and enjoy vast improvements in their quality of life. Neurofeedback training got my life back on track, and I'm thankful that I am now able to make the same difference for others.

Should you try neurofeedback training? I can't say definitively before the evaluation that it will be right for you or your child. What I can tell you is that, in so many ways, brain-based disorders can wreak havoc, both on the lives of the people who suffer from them and on the lives of their loved ones. For many of my patients, neurofeedback training has brought hope where no hope had existed.

A Final Thought

I'm confident neurofeedback training can help you. I know it won't hurt you. And I'm happy and excited that you've read this book, because it gave me an opportunity to share with you how neurofeedback training helped me, and how it can give you or your loved ones a healthier brain and a better life!

Thank you for reading this. Let me know if my staff and I can be of service!

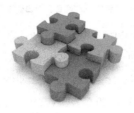

Resources for Readers on Neurofeedback Training

Carlton Neurofeedback Center

For residents of the greater Washington, D.C. area, the Carlton Neurofeedback Center is located in Manassas, Virginia, and you are welcome to call us to set up an appointment for a free initial evaluation. Our Website is full of articles and research about neurofeedback training and its effective use for specific brain-based disorders. You may visit our Website to further explore neurofeedback training, view videos, or schedule a free evaluation for you or a family member.

Carlton Neurofeedback Center
8805 Sudley Road, Suite 200, Manassas, VA 20110
Telephone: (703) 335-9149
Website: http://www.carltonneurofeedbackcenter.com/

Find a Certified Neurofeedback Center Near You

The nonprofit organization which certifies neurofeedback and biofeedback providers in the United States and around the world is the Biofeedback Certification International Alliance (BCIA). The BCIA Website lets you search for certified neurofeedback providers in your area and provides both contact and credential information. The Website has a helpful "Find a Practitioner" tab where you can enter your location and receive a list of providers. *Look for the letters BCN,* indicating a board-certified neurofeedback provider.

Biofeedback Certification International Alliance
Website: www.BCIA.org

For Further Information and Research on Neurofeedback

If you'd like to dig deeper to learn more about neurofeedback training, you may visit the Website of the International Society for Neurofeedback and Research. This membership organization provides a wealth of in-depth information about neurofeedback, including research, articles, media coverage, and a wide variety of resources.

International Society for Neurofeedback and Research
Website: www.isnr.org

CPSIA information can be obtained
at www.ICGtesting.com
Printed in the USA
FSOW04n0429031017
39441FS